A MODERN GUIDE TO HATS

Written & illustrated
by Steve Harris

Nightingale
*An imprint of Wimbledon Publishing Company
London*

Copyright © 2000
Illustrations © 2000 WPC

First published in Great Britain in 2000
by Wimbledon Publishing Company Ltd
P.O. Box 9779 London SW19 7ZG
All rights reserved

First published 2000 in Great Britain

ISBN: 1903222 01 X

Produced in Great Britain
Printed and bound in Hungary

> *'Death wears a big hat
> 'Coz He's a big bloke'*
>
> — Elvis Costello

INTRODUCTION

by Dame Margot Geauxgo,
Professor of Millinery History,
All Sods College, Cambridge.

As a little girl, I'd go with my family to church on Sundays - sellotaped into my best hat. It was like a religion with us. I stared up at Christ in His bowler and my passion was born.

During the War strict rationing forced us to wear powdered egg. Where my mother's favourite bonnet once stood, there is now a council estate. And if I'd had this book when I was doing my PhD, I could have finished in half the time, and arrived unflustered at the Ambassador's reception. Never dip your hat into International Fondue. Bah.

Dame M. Geauxgo
1999

FEDORA

Characteristics: low, soft felt hat with lengthwise crease in the crown.

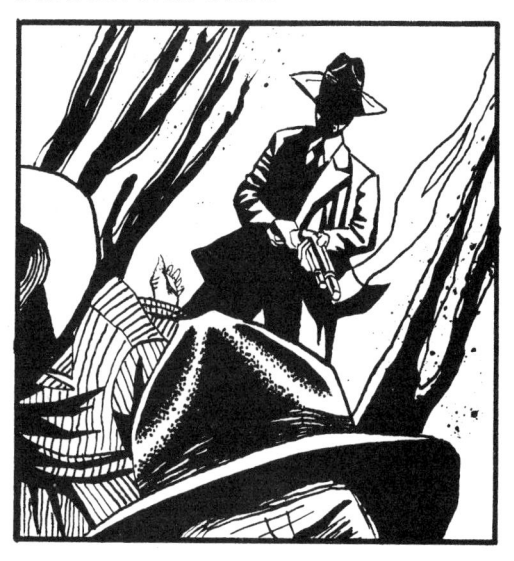

In the heady days of prohibition, to wear a fedora was to declare, 'I am a vicious mobster', which is why, in a lightning piece of judicial genius, New York State outlawed the hat overnight. The next day saw the arrests of over 100 hoodlums - including Al Capone for 'possession with intent to wear'. The crime scene responded swiftly: failed pickpocket turned underworld supremo, Elbows McGinty, pioneered the wearing of armbands with 'I am a vicious mobster' printed in very small type to evade detection by a blinkered police force.

Despite the repealing of the law in 1935, the fedora wouldn't be seen again in any number until the early Eighties when female New Romantic pop singers wore them mercilessly. Public outcry demanded a return of the ban but none was forthcoming.

CYCLING HELMET
Characteristics: punk tortoise.

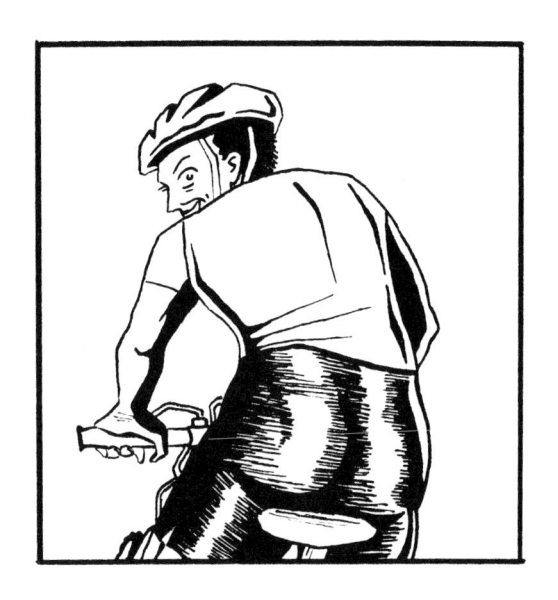

Early Victorian cycling helmets were steam powered, noisy and cumbersome and nobody wore them. Thus it remained for over a century.

In the post-industrial 1980's, cycling deaths began to increase sharply as drivers lost control laughing at new skin-tight cycling shorts. The helmet returned as a means of diverting attention from lycra clad buttocks. Initial designs were mushroom-like, prompting unfounded fears that they were nuclear powered. In a desperate attempt to claw back some credibility, the current streamlined shape evolved, although some cyclists still hide behind masks in embarrassment. Despite on-going worries about exhaust emissions, the cycling helmet remains the safest piece of equipment to wear whilst falling under the wheels of a juggernaut.

CLOCHE HAT

Characteristics: close-fitting, bell-shaped hat.

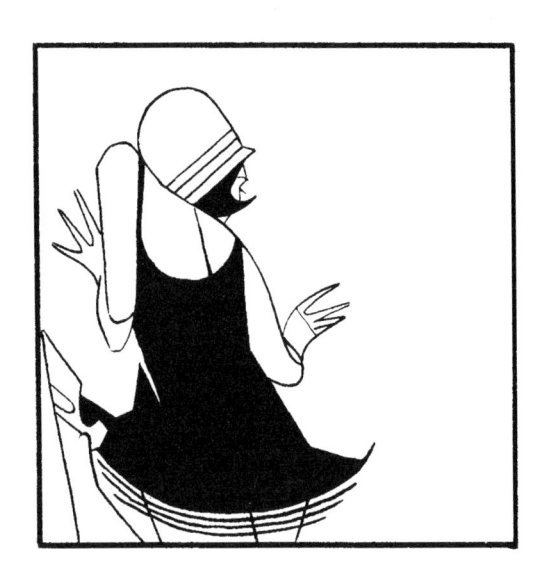

In the Twenties, women started wearing trousers and denying their curves in very straight dresses. Hair was worn short and angular. Through mathematical precision lay a form of freedom and there was no greater exponent of this than the flapper in her cloche hat. A snug helmet, the cloche fitted perfectly over the bob like a travelling case for the head, showing off the beautiful curves of the cranium rather than the body. With its overtones of sexual ambiguity complementing the gender-bending mood of the era, the Catholic Church were preparing to ban the cloche hat when Pope Omnibus the 67th took to wearing one and performing the Charleston through the Vatican, blessing the people with his heels.

BOBBLE HAT

Characteristics: close-fitting, dome-shaped hat surmounted by a pom-pom.

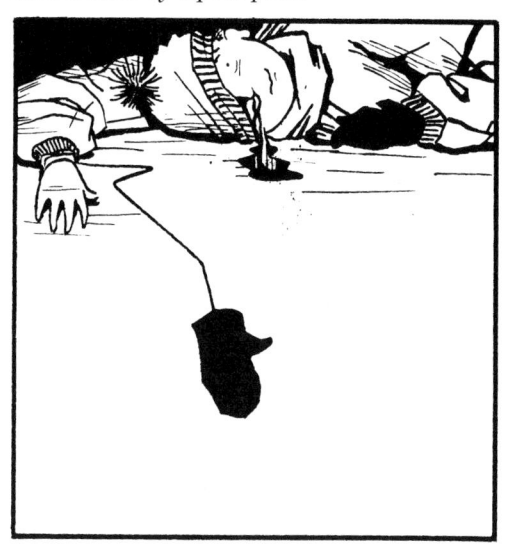

In 1645 the Cavaliers took a winter break from the rigours of the English civil war on the fashionable ski slopes of Europe. Adapting the established woollen bonnet to their own flamboyant style, the bobble hat quickly established itself as de rigeur winter wear, combining warm practicality with a jaunty flourish. But although the pom-pom seems a devil-may-care gesture, it later found cruel use in the hands of the playground bully as a handy grip with which to bang the wearer's head on the ground.

Sadly, with modern puritanical sophistication, this hat is a much derided form of headgear. If they don't take it upon themselves, wearers may undergo forced bobblectomy by an angry mob.

BENNY HAT

Characteristics: a bobble hat that's all hat and no bobble.

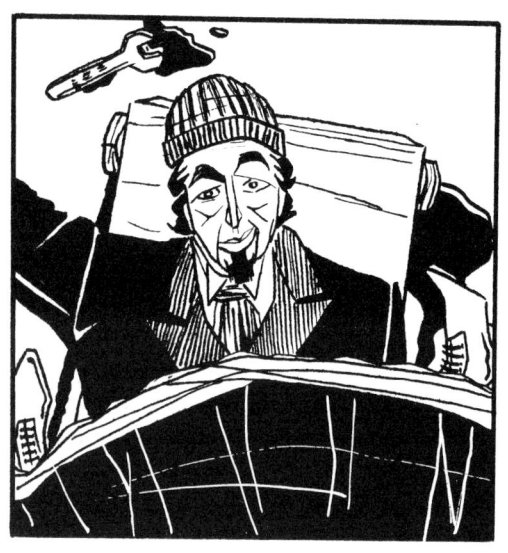

Ever the sensible older brother of the bobble hat, the Benny hat has been worn chiefly by mechanics and sappers, a sober association stemming from its invention by Benjamin Disraeli (1804-81). Wishing to keep the grease from his hair during one of Queen Victoria's routine oil changes, Disraeli found to hand a bobble hat. Tactfully pruning the pom-pom as a mark of respect for his mechanical monarch he gave birth to the functional and versatile working hat which came to be called, 'Benny'.

Today the hat is a stylistically, indeed morally, acceptable alternative to its pompommed sibling, adopted by the earnest everywhere from fashion police, to social workers, to eco-warriors. A resounding triumph for the roundheads.

ASCOT

Characteristics: extravagantly ludicrous hats of varying style worn for racing at Royal Ascot.

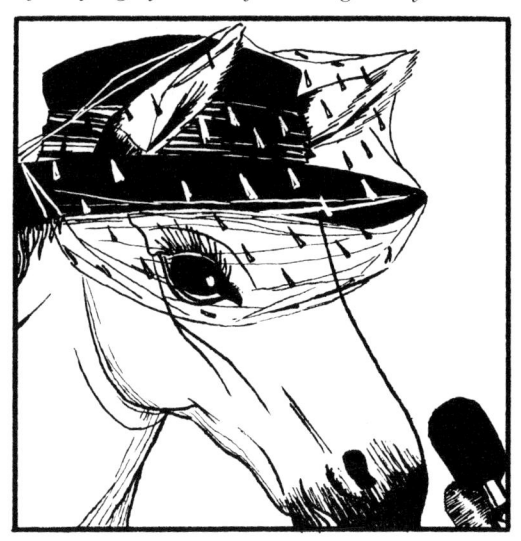

No one is sure when horses started wearing hats while racing at Royal Ascot, but what the tradition lacks in safety, it more than makes up for in spectacle. The sight of thoroughbreds thundering down the course in eye-boggling millinery creations has been likened to the mothers' egg and spoon race on sports day at Eton.

Always controversial, animal rights campaigners say that horses were never meant to wear hats. This claim was somewhat scuppered by the 1980 favourite, Daily Snortgrind, who veered off the track - while leading by a nose - to start a successful TV career. Extremely popular, Ms Snortgrind still wears superior hats and produces better manure than most of her talk-show contemporaries.

BASEBALL CAP

Characteristics: generously-proportioned cap with a peak.

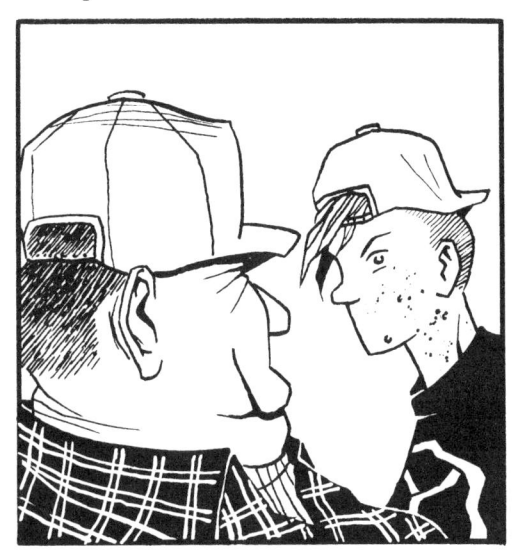

The baseball cap is the hat which came to embody the American dream. With a one-size-fits-all mentality, and ample room on the front for logos and advertising, its heart will always be Stateside. There, entire hoardings have been built on baseball caps, and they are worn by judges, the FBI, the homeless, and Barbara Bush. With thousands of uses, it may not be long before somebody works out what they are.

A recent twist in the style of the baseball cap has been to reverse it; the inquisitive will always want a 'peak round the back' and an adjustable gusset at the front. Shrewdly spotting this niche in the market, hat companies spent millions retooling to produce the reverse cap. A credulous public now buys both kinds.

BOWLER HAT

Characteristics: dome-shaped, hard felt hat with narrow, turned-up brim.

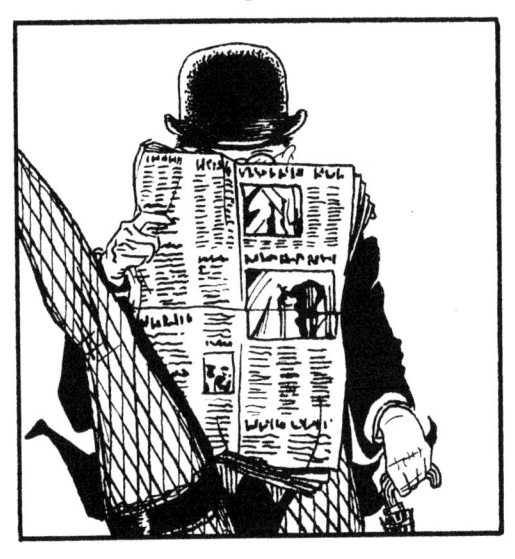

A British bank is built on tradition. Tradition is built on a black bowler hat. Although the bowler has been superseded in turn by slick hair and hands-free mobile phone technology, it was for years the staple head piece in the City of London.

A City scene: bowler hats at five p.m. worn above spectacles, neat moustaches, tail coats, fish net stockings, high heels. The air is filled with clicking as high kicking bank clerks mildly meander their way through rain shiny streets to railway stations, destination suburban idyll in the Suspender Belt; ginger cats, maiden aunts, baths full of Robinsons marmalade.

TEN GALLON HAT

Characteristics: large-brimmed hat with a tall crown.

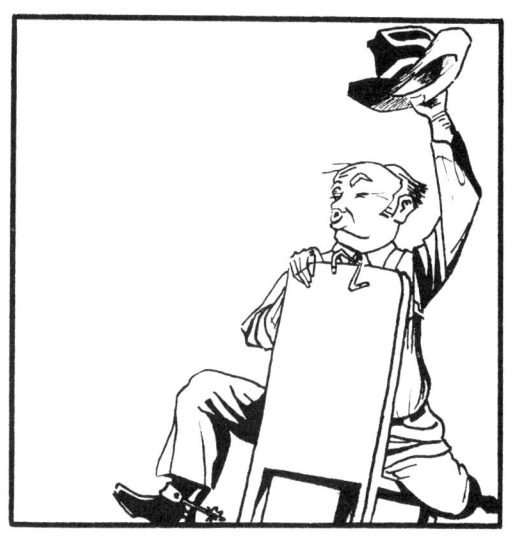

The ten gallon hat can take a little over three pints in liquid, which is under half a gallon - slightly less in shrimp. However, using the hat as a receptacle for any amount of liquid or seafood renders it difficult to wear.

Known also as the stetson, the tall crown of the ten gallon was useful in gunfights for misleading opponents as to the exact whereabouts of the head. However, since the outlawing of weapons for cattle in 1974, modern cowboys have led a peaceful life and now wear small tassel-less fezzes, sometimes with a pretty veil. This leaves Texan businessmen to do all the stetson wearing. As evidence shows they can withstand direct shots to the head, with no effect other than impaired eyesight, their choice of hat must be attributed to lack of judgement.

EASTER BONNET

Characteristics: an up-turned flower basket.

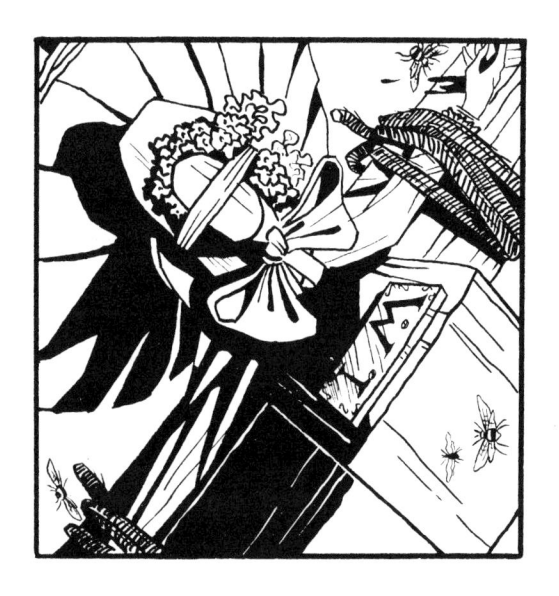

The Easter bonnet takes as its form the traditional Sunday bonnet, but is festooned to celebrate the Christian festival of Easter. Around the turn of the century, fashionable middle class women would compete to display the most elaborate bonnet decorations at Easter Sunday church parades and picnics. What started with flowers, fruit, potato salad and ribbons ended with scale models of Calvary in wicker; and life sized crucifixes:

'Mrs Piminy Geribald of Cheroot Gardens, posing on the crucifix in her own hat, won great praise for her realistic raspberry jam stigmata, but was later fatally stung by a wasp.'
-St. Jive Gazette, Easter 1902.

These hats served as a reminder that Easter is a time of hope, rebirth and neck-braces.

HOODS

Characteristics: a headpiece attached to another garment, usually a coat, rarely trousers.

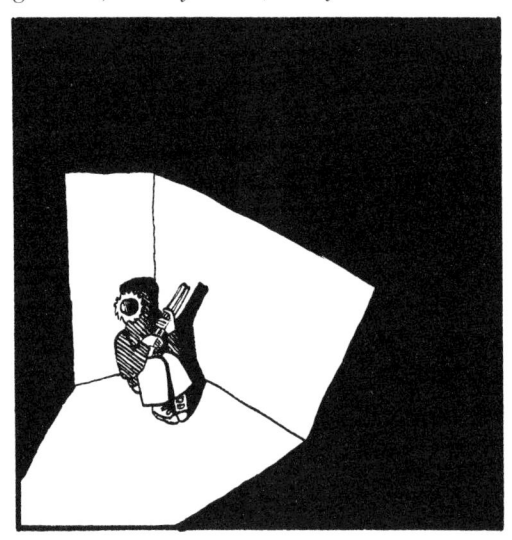

Since Little Red Riding Hood's archetypal cowl, the hood has protected the innocent from the horrors of the outside world. However, limited peripheral vision can lead to paranoia and spiralling fear. Should this happen, the snorkel hood of the parka jacket is the best place to hide. Acting as a portable cave, it is a place of warmth and retreat. Children have been known to don their parkas never to be seen again, either through their total concealment, or because of a brutal zip.

Conversely, since Little Black Death's apocalyptic cowl, the hood has also concealed the face of Evil. Today's urban terrorist favours the elfin jogging top, grabbing the hood by its drawstrings to pull it screaming into the dark alley of modern life; a fairy tale violation of innocence.

TOP HAT
Characteristics: silk hat with a tall, flat-topped crown.

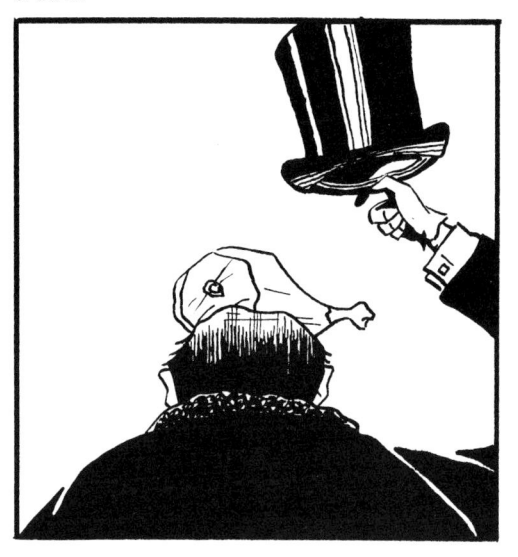

Grey for morning dress, shiny and black at night, the top hat has always been a place where a gentleman could discreetly conceal a ham. Opera hats came in collapsible models, and the taller the hat, the more likely it was to collapse. They were eventually banned after the Venice Opera House tragedy of 1898. Twenty-three people were killed when the nine foot hat of one Arturo Flaminzi fell from the lethal height of the upper circle, showering the audience below with fatal sides of mutton, beef, and sherry trifle with which he'd planned to see out one of the lengthier arias.

Seen these days only at weddings, and the more amusing funerals, the silk topper will be best remembered as Fred Astaire's dancing partner in films such as *Brisket! Brisket!* (1935)

RASTAFARIAN HAT

Characteristics: woollen hat of amorphous shape in the coloured stripes of the Ethiopian flag.

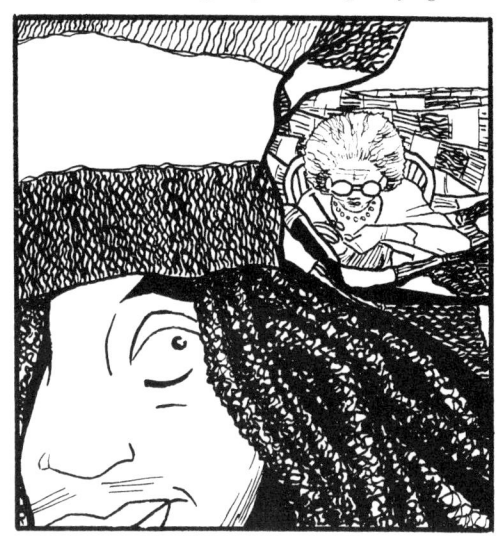

The white bourgeois offspring of the sold-out, drop-out, flower-power generation, wear their Kangol Rastafarian hats at a rakish angle to display the black roots in their blond dreadlocks. These lost Children of the Cause like to get stoned and dream about being oppressed, while watching *Selassie Come Home* (1943).

In fact, real Rastafarian hats are only knitted by real Jamaican grandmothers, who won't sell out for less than a cup of herbal tea and a box of cheap cigars. The hats range in size and shape from beret to windsock, the latter caused by 'knitting frenzy', where dozens of venerable old women pile into a scrum, frantically knitting one garment between them for as long as anyone will throw them wool and food.

TRILBY

Characteristics: soft felt hat with a turned-up brim at the back and a length-wise crease in the crown.

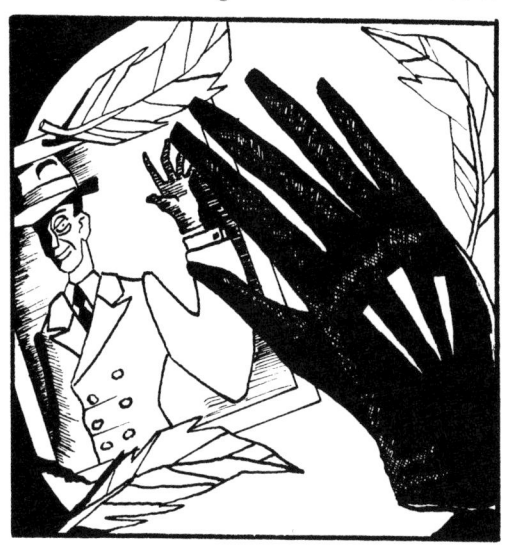

Trilby was a respectable, smart young hat about town between the wars. Great chums with the vivacious Pigskin-Glove twins, they were often seen gadding about in open topped motor cars, out of which Trilby was blown several times.

Passed over for service in WWII, Trilby declined into a life of black-market racketeering, teaming up with Spiv Moustache and Feather Boa. By the late Sixties, Spiv had been fatally slashed with a razor, and Feather was plucked. A stained, raddled Trilby pulled himself together. One best-selling book of amusing underworld anecdotes later, he was back on his feet. Elderly now, he has regained his charm and still has them laughing in the old hats' home.

FLY FISHERMAN'S HAT

Characteristics: like a floppy-brimmed lampshade.

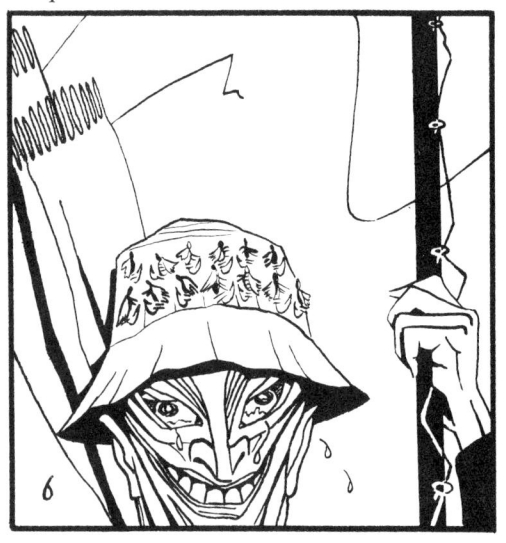

Fisherman may keep their fishing flies stuck in their hat, but if they're wise, they hook them in when the hat is off. It is so easy to pierce the scalp, effectively stitching the hat to the head, and this is why inexperienced fishermen always seem to grin in a high wind.

In the last decade, the fisherman's hat has become an item of cool, worn first by rappers in khaki trousers and plimsolls, then by neo-mods in khaki trousers and plimsolls. A fresh trout is optional in either case. The overall look is one of laid back hip that's so mellow it's positively boring.

BALACLAVA

Characteristics: close-fitting head-covering with a hole left for the face.

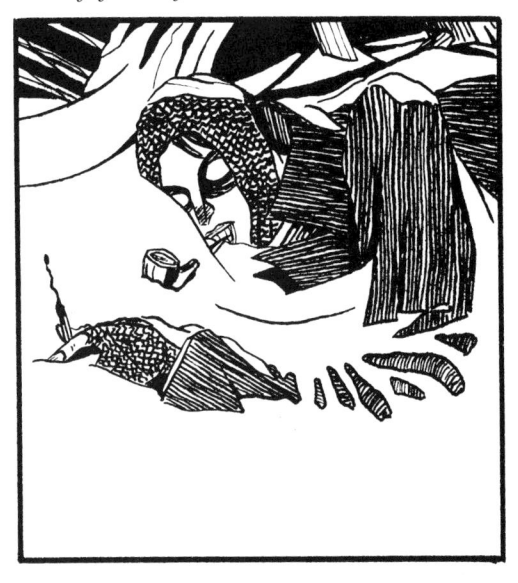

It was during the Crimean War (1853-56) that the Balaclava helmet was invented by the Queen's Own Darners (motto: To Darn or Be Darned Trying). With all round cranial coverage it became a very popular piece of winter woollenry, although many British soldiers still used pipes to keep their lips warm on the battlefield.

The advent of a dark period for the balaclava came with a refinement of the design which aimed to increase coverage. Instead of one large hole, three small ones were left for eyes and mouth only. This version has been adopted by terrorists and bank robbers who strike fear into their victims' hearts with their uncanny resemblance to bowling balls.

FLAT CAP

Characteristics: snug-fitting cap with small, recessed peak.

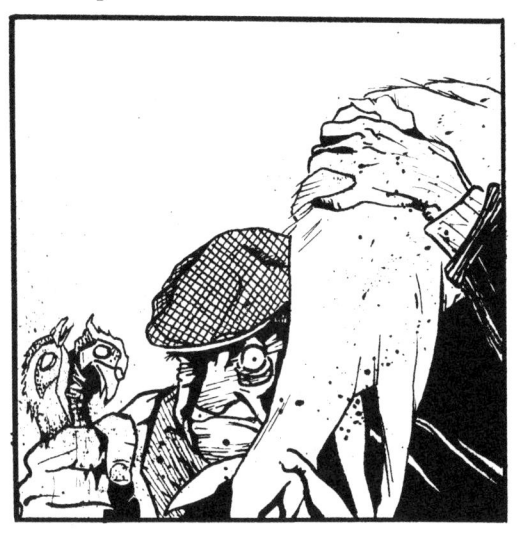

Bred in northern England for use by gamekeepers, the flat cap found favour with common men and the gentry alike. Dogged, versatile and loyal, it is very much a chap's cap and makes an excellent working hat. The decline in both heavy and countryside industries has seen flat cap numbers dwindle; they are distinctly mediocre pets and are bred mainly for illegal fighting now. Not a vicious hat, but tenacious, the flat cap has been known to outlast fierce Russian fur hats, preserving stamina with short sharp attacks to the ear flaps. Recent cross breeding with its cousin, the golfing retriever, has produced a soft, pastel coloured flat cap. Though a betrayal of its working roots, this fashionable upstart could be the only future for a tough little hat.

PANAMA

Characteristics: narrow-brimmed hat of straw made from pine leaves.

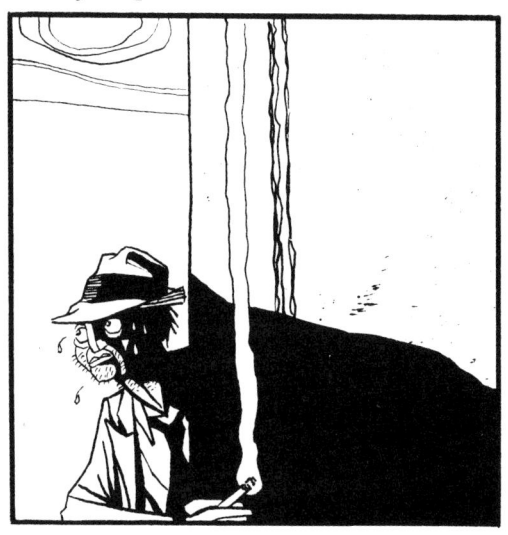

Havana tobacco-leaf smoking hat, the Panama is close but no cigar. Arguably the quintessential hat for the Englishman abroad in hot climates, it is certainly smarter than the knotted hanky or the sombrero and is best worn with a crisp linen suit in a little light salad dressing. Anything less than crisp will not do, unless very creased and dirty, accessorised with four days' greasy stubble and a haunted look.

Englishmen should never don the Panama at home; those that do have a filthy habit of wearing blazers and replacing the hat's black band with an old school tie. If one must do this, take care to remove the schoolboy from the tie first, modern parents are very litigious.

BRETTON FISHERMAN'S CAP

Characteristics: semi-aquatic, flattish, round cap with small, semi-circular peak.

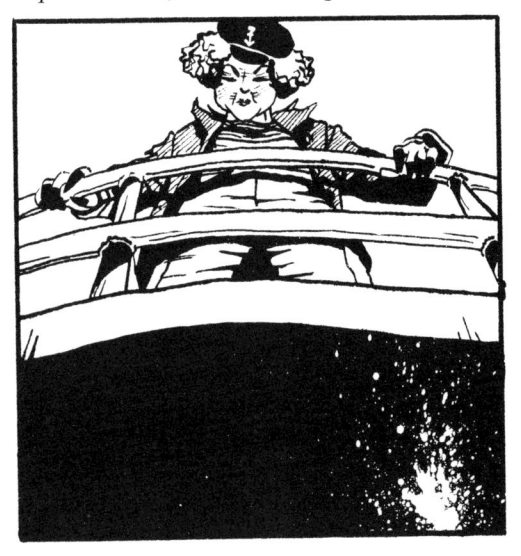

The eponymous cap of the Bretton fisherman is a strangely schizophrenic creature. It spends much of its time lying on the fisherman's salt encrusted head, or warding off lecherous barnacles. The cap vies for territory with the roll-up fag (distant relation of the roll mop herring) that lives symbiotically behind the fisherman's ear.

The cap's other habitat is high up in the wind swept curls of rich yacht dwellers, where it nests precariously above vistas of blazer and black-and-white striped T-shirts. The cap survives here by imitating its rustic brother. Quite how it is possible to look rustic on a £2 million motor boat is unclear, but the yacht dwellers seem unconcerned.

SOMBRERO

Characteristics: wide-brimmed, straw hat with a round crown.

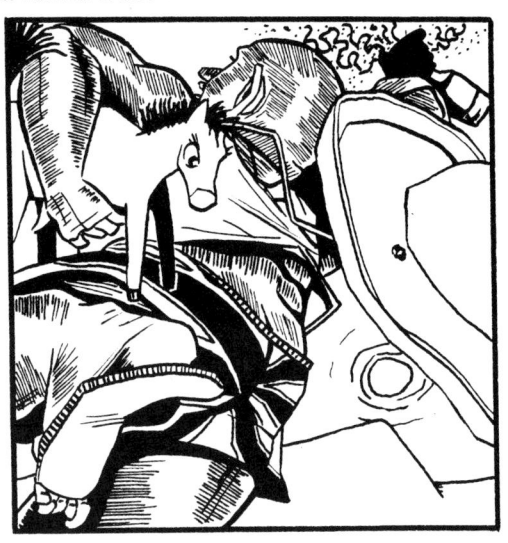

The wide brim of the sombrero serves two purposes: to shade the wearer from the sun during the day, and to support a sheet of canvas at night, providing an impromptu tent for the ultimate in mobile homes. Modern sombreros come with foundations, a damp course, running water, and some luxury versions even have a heli-pad, but purists feel this is all missing the point somewhat.

Also missing the point are the British holiday makers who bring back sombreros from anywhere sunny and foreign, neglecting to don their protective headgear until they are on the plane home, thus achieving a startling crimson colour with which to entertain their friends.

STRAW BOATER

Characteristics: round, flat-topped straw hat with wide, flat brim.

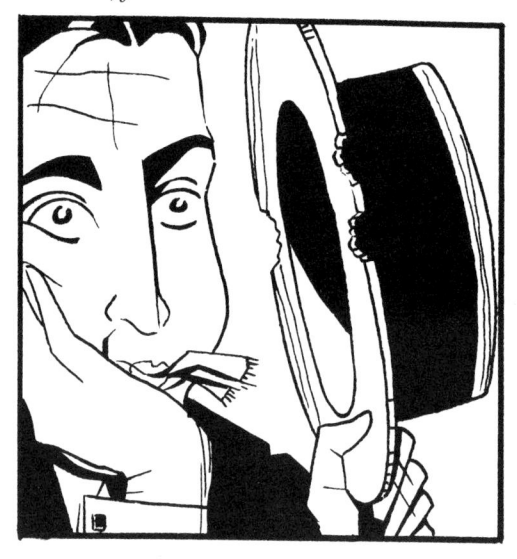

Worn by natty, dapper dandies in the first half of the twentieth century, the straw boater was light and carefree, a hat that could be eaten between meals without spoiling your appetite. A sure sign of a young man's success was the absence of teeth marks in the brim of his boater. That brim could cause problems, but Chovis P. Nub had a novel solution in his *Handbook for Chaps* (1922): 'Write an informative or witty message in your hat. Should you inadvertently lean against a wall, thus causing your boater to stand erect, you will amuse and entertain passers-by without looking a fool.'

This backfired for one poor fellow who wrote the factually correct 'Valentino smells of horseradish', and was lynched where he stood.

SUMMER HAT

Characteristics: light, wide-brimmed hat of varying style.

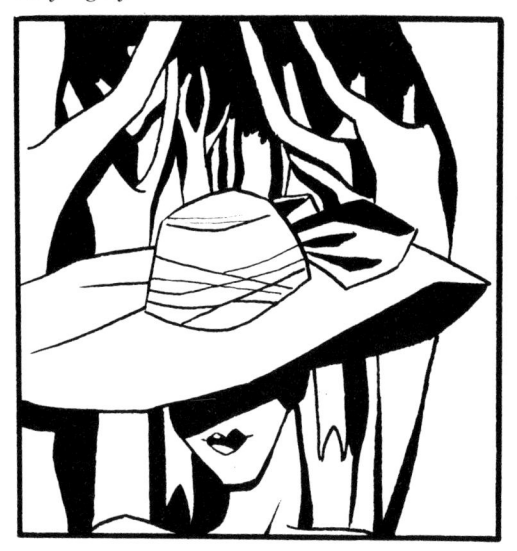

Summer is a mythical time in England, and female summer hats evoke romantic, pastoral images of its countryside. The troubled poet laureate Jayson F'Arson penned his *'Ode to Summers Passed'* after his divorce from Rubella Trefwthick in 1951:

When you wear your summer hat
Your face becomes a bower,
With brows where nymphs and fawns have sat.
And nostrils where I shower.

Your mouth becomes a babbling stream
Whose ripples softly glimmer.
It's stocked with trout and perch and bream,
I've caught one for my dinner.

But with no hat a harlot shows
Turning elves to traitors,
Nymphs and fawns becoming nympho-
Maniacs and fornicators.

FEZ

Characteristics: small, brimless, flat-topped conical hat, with a tassel.

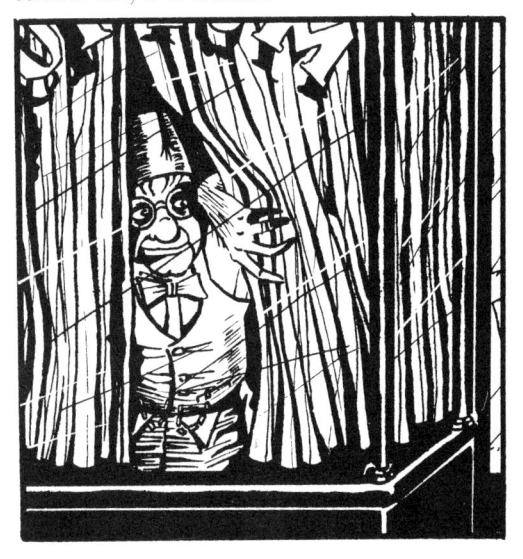

During the drug-crazed nineteenth century, opium suppliers noticed that their drab and ordinary salesmen were robbing the drug of its mystique; a change of image was needed. As if by magic, the fez appeared. Transforming grey opium clerks into pointless wizards, the fez was at once ridiculous and sinister and full of Eastern promise. (Note: of course, in the East the fez is an everyday hat. When they wish to look sinister and ridiculous there, they write the word 'muffin' on their heads.)

Opium parlours and emporia, where people could dress up and indulge in hallucinogenic fantasies, did marvellous business thanks to the fez. Then someone invented fondue and the spell was broken.

THE FEMALE TURBAN

Characteristics: a long stripe of material wrapped several times around the head.

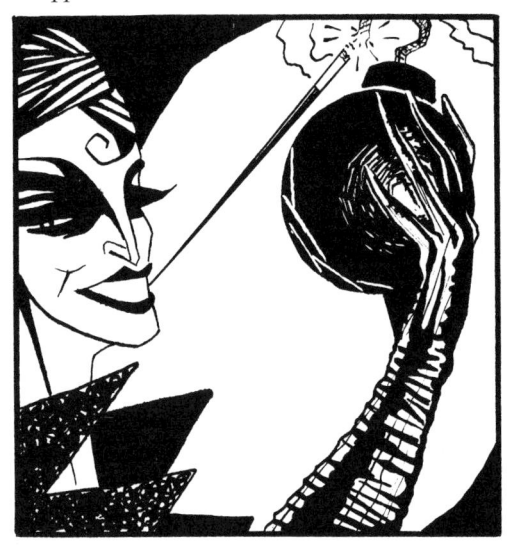

A perennial favourite with bohemian naso-swarvines robed in flowing dakmuts and fogmereens, the female turban found glamour with femme fatales and spies, like Manita Twengo, the devastatingly sexy hod-carrier-turned-double-agent.

It is now largely a domestic headpiece, fashioned from a towel to dry the hair. However, intrigue and scandal still lurk nearby; recent times have seen an increasing number of deaths by turban. Inexperienced men apparently try to emulate their wives, tying perfect turbans but starting too low, suffocating in their own cocoon. Even bald men have fallen foul of this phenomenon, a fact which the police have deemed to be 'merely circumstantial'. Are these unfortunate husbands really just the victims of 'tragic accidents'?

BERET

Characteristics: round, flattish hat with the remains of its stalk.

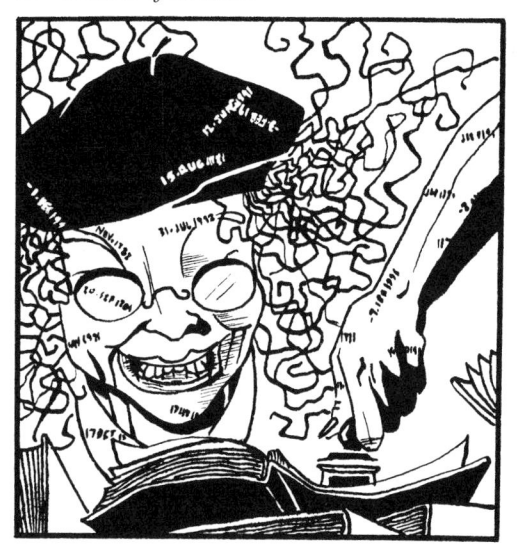

The beret isn't, as the name suggests, a berry, but a gourd. Grown in the stink groves of southern Europe, the beret is harvested in August and hollowed of its smelly pulp, which is then trodden and fermented to make hair lacquer. Meanwhile, the leathery skins are shipped north to mature and soften on the heads of beat poets in the beer cellars of Paris and Berlin.

Associated irretrievably in the public consciousness with Frenchmen and onions, the beret is, in fact, almost exclusively worn by the mackintoshed librarians of Wiltshire and Berkshire.

CARMEN MIRANDA

Characteristics: a fruit barrow mounted on a woman's turban.

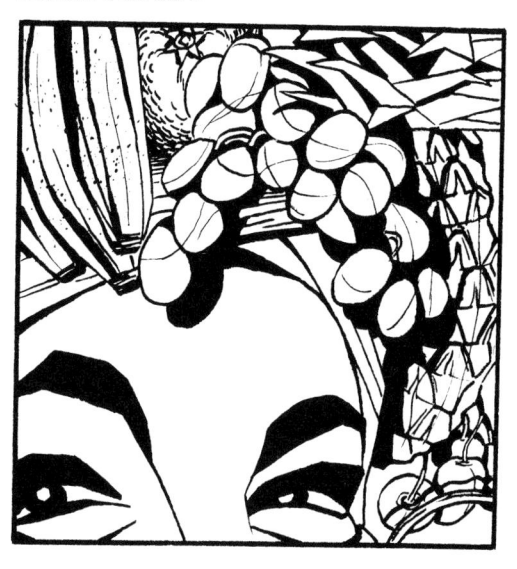

Although something of a one off, the woman with the tutti-frutti hat lives on in the public memory. Having achieved little success and severe back pain as 'the woman with the pooper-scooper hat', Cuban film goddess Carmen Miranda (1909-1955) took the opportunity to reinvent herself with a brilliant satire on the American Pineapple Crisis in the film musical *Ay-ay-ay-ay-ay-ay-ay-ay Ananas Comosus* (1946). The resulting fashion craze lasted as long as it took people to tire of buying a fresh hat every few days, but saved the fledgling pineapple industry.

RIDING HAT

Characteristics: dome-shaped felt covered helmet, with a small peak.

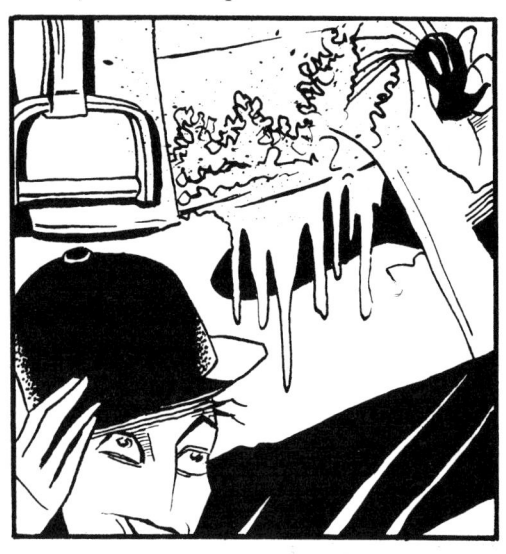

Ostensibly a protective helmet, the riding hat is inextricably linked with fetishism and images of shiny leather boots, horses in jodhpurs, whips, severely tailored jackets, and the kinky sport of dressage in which riders race to cover their mount in vinaigrette using a shaving brush.

It is no surprise to learn that this all started with a depraved handful of the English upper classes, but they are the minority. Every day horse riders respectably go about their business of trampling on peasants, ravaging stable boys, and terrorising milk maids, with none of the sordid nonsense described above. And, in their trusty riding hats, they have no fear of head injury when the rocks start flying.

HEADSCARF

Characteristics: take one large square of material folded diagonally, and divide the classes with it.

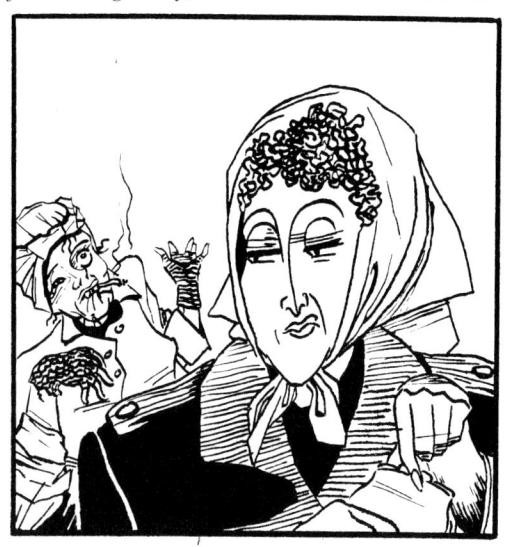

Nipping out to the supermarket in 1978, the Queen's headscarf came undone and the middle classes held their breath. In a trice, ten Household Cavalrymen were upon her, retying it under the chin. With the peak of the triangle pulled into place at her neck, they gently replaced her crown and the headscarf was safe.

Had they tied the knot at the forehead, pulled the peak over the hair, tucked it under and back over the knot, the Cavalrymen would have created the char or landlady of popular legend. The addition of a floral apron and a droopy fag hanging from lower lip, and Britain would have had a gossiping old biddy for Sovereign. On such a thread does the monarchy hang.